The Autoimmune Diet

Nourishing Your True Identity

With Meals That Heal

by

Anne Angelone

TABLE OF CONTENT

THE AUTOIMMUNE DIET 0
Copyright © by Anne Angelone 2013 1
Introduction 2
Guidelines 5

FOODS TO INCLUDE: 7
Fruits 7
Vegetables 7
Dense carbs 7
Fungi 7
Wild fish 8
Meat 8
Milk and yogurt 8
Fats 8
Coconut 8
Beverages 8
Teas 9
Fermented foods 9
Condiments 9
Herbs and spices 9
Sugar substitutes 9

FOODS TO ELIMINATE: 10
Nightshade vegetables 10
Fruit 10
Processed and canned meats 10
Fish 10
Nuts and Seeds 10
Dairy 11
Oils 11
Beans and Legumes 11
Fungi 11
Soy 11
Drinks 11
Condiments 11
Sweeteners 12
Grains 12
Grain products 12
Grain like substances or pseudo-cereals 12
Gluten containing foods 12
Legumes 13
Lectins 13

Dairy 13
Eggs: 13
Alcohol 13
All processed food 13
Sugars 13
Seed based spices 13
Berry and fruit based spices 14
Coffee 14
Tea 14
Avoid immune stimulants 14
A word about Caution foods 14

CONSIDERATIONS: 15
FODMAPs 15
FODMAPs in the AIP 15
SIBO caution foods in the Autoimmune Diet 16

REINTRODUCTION OF FOODS: 17
Avoid immune stimulants: 17

DELICIOUS RECIPES: 18
Green smoothies 18
Veggie stew 18
Coconut Yogurt 19
Kale Chips 19
Grill Pan Chicken 19
Tri-Tip Steak and Asparagus 20
Coconut Chicken Paillard 20
Braised Greens 20
Carmelized Brussels Sprouts 21
Baked Tilapia with Lemon and Fresh Herbs 21
Super greens salad 22
Ginger avo coco dressing 22
Basic Beef Bone Broth 22
Ginger root tea: 23
Arugula Salad With Grilled Tri Tip 23
Pan Seared yellowtail witH sauteed Rainbow chard 24
Chicken Vegetable Soup 24
Tuna steaks with Sauteed spinach 25
NEw York Steak and Salad 25
Steamed Halibut with sauteed greens 26
Stir fried Chicken breast with zucchini, avocado and basil 26
Turmeric Chicken with zucchini 27
Rosemary baked Lamb Chops on a bed of Kale Chips 27
Balsamic marinated pork chops with mashed turnips and sauteed

- collards 28
- Crock pot chicken 28
- Grill pan pork chops..29
- Zucchini Pasta with seasoned ground beef 29
- Bacon Wrapped Chicken Thighs 30
- Rosemary Rubbed Cornish Hens 30
- Ground turkey Breakfast Sautee 31
- Ahi tuna with sauteed red chard 31
- Carrot ginger Soup..32
- Grass Fed Beef burger 32
- Tri Tip with sauteed Greens and Mashed Cauliflower.........................33
- Grilled Chicken breast with Bright Green Olives 33
- Rib eye steak with sauteed swiss chard and sweet potato fries 34
- Sweet potato fries 34
- Pacific Snapper with lemon, Thyme and Capers 34
- Chicken stock..35
- Shrimp Sauteed with bok Choy 35
- Grilled Balsamic Pork Tenderloin...35
- Cilantro Roast Chicken..36
- Garlic Rosemary Salmon...36
- Beef Stew..37
- Sautéed Kale...37
- Ginger Salmon and Broccoli 37
- Nori Chips 38
- Porterhouse steak with kale and avocado 38
- Spaghetti squash with ground Turkey, greens and artichoke hearts .39
- Lemon orange Clay pot chicken..40

- DESSERTS 41
- Coconut berry ice cream 41
- Raspberries with coconut milk and balsamic vinegar........................41
- Snack ideas: 41
- Detox Support: Transitioning to The Autoimmune Diet....................42
- Detox Broth: 42

- ADDITIONAL DETOX SUPPORT..43
- Liver Detox:..43
- Raw Apple Cider Vinegar: 43
- Reducing Stress and Improving Sleep...43

- FINAL THOUGHTS 44
- ABOUT THE AUTHOR 45
- Autoimmune Paleo resources: 46

COPYRIGHT © BY ANNE ANGELONE 2013 ALL RIGHTS RESERVED

No part of this publication may be reproduced in any form or by any means, including scanning, photocopying, or otherwise without prior written permission of the copyright holder.

ISBN-13: **978-1489553577**
ISBN-10: **1489553576**

Disclaimer

This program manual is not intended to provide medical advice or to take the place of medical advice and treatment from your personal physician

Readers are advised to consult their own doctors or other qualified health professionals regarding the treatment of medical conditions

The author, shall not be held liable or responsible for any misunderstanding or misuse of the information contained in this program manual or for any loss, damage, or injury caused or alleged to be caused directly or indirectly by any treatment, action, or application of any food or food source discussed in this program manual

The statements in this program manual have not been evaluated by the U.S Food and Drug Administration

This information is not intended to diagnose, treat, cure, or prevent any disease.

To request permission for reproduction or inquire about consulting about autoimmunity, please contact:

Anne Angelone, Licensed Acupuncturist

website: www.anneangelone.com

INTRODUCTION

This guide will help you avoid the most irritating foods for autoimmune conditions.

The goal of The Autoimmune Diet is to fix your leaky gut and eliminate food and bacterial triggers to autoimmune reactions with the ultimate intention of decreasing your flare-ups and severity of autoimmune attacks

The Autoimmune Diet is designed to rapidly reduce inflammation and heal intestinal permeability via specific dietary interventions. To calm down the immune/inflammatory response and allow the gut to fully heal, you will need to remove the major offending foods: eggs, grains, alcohol, nightshades, nuts, seeds, legumes, and dairy.

For anyone with an autoimmune disease, eliminating known inflammatory foods from your diet, resolving dysbiosis, and healing the mucosal lining of the small intestine are the keys to optimal health and balanced immunity.

While on the The Autoimmune Diet, it is important to identify and remove overgrowths of yeast, bacteria and parasites that may also be driving your immune/inflammatory response. The goal of the autoimmune diet is to increase anti-inflammatory and probiotic foods to heal the integrity of the gut lining while simultaneously eliminating the foods that create low grade immune/inflammatory responses, irritate the gut lining, and feed harmful bacteria By eliminating the underlying mechanisms that drive inflammation and autoimmunity, you can modulate and bring balance to your overactive immune system.

It may be a new lens through which to consider how poorly digested foods continue to irritate the lining of your gut, feed your yeast and bacterial overgrowths, trigger autoantibody responses, and may set the stage for you to express your genetic tendency to autoimmunity. Yet, since 60- 80% of your immune system is in your gut, you probably already know that digestive health is of paramount importance in healing autoimmune conditions.

You will be utilizing a nutrient dense, plant strong nutritional model designed to remove foods that activate immune responses, irritate the gut lining, and contribute to leaky gut. After 30 days on this plan you should notice significant health benefits. Some will need to continue strictly on this plan for 1 year or longer before any potential food triggers can be introduced. The Autoimmune diet is encouraged as a safe way of decreasing inflammation in your body and helping to heal your leaky gut. Following the "foods to include" list will supply you with nutrient dense, bioavailable vitamins and minerals. Your immune system and genes will be shored up with the right nutrition, allowing your inflamed gut to begin healing.

Exercising for 30 minutes a day is a natural anti-inflammatory and is encouraged for balanced immune function and enhanced sleep.

Other significant considerations for autoimmune conditions include resolving dysbiosis, supporting detoxification and methylation, ramping up glutathione, and increasing regulatory T-cells with vitamin D, probiotics, and fish oils.

All of this will go a long way to reduce inflammation and balance the immune system.

The Autoimmune Diet is inspired by successful treatment outcomes in applying Nutrigenomics, Functional Medicine, Dr Kharazzian's RepairVite program and the Paleo Autoimmune Protocol. Many thanks to Elaine Fawcett and Sarah Ballantyne, PhD for help in writing, editing and getting the word out about nutrition for autoimmune conditions.

I would like to dedicate this project to everyone navigating an autoimmune disorder. Stay cool and learn how to keep your immune/inflammatory response at an all time low.

GUIDELINES

Do's

- Eat organic, pastured, grass fed animal protein and wild fish.
- Eat carbohydrates from fruits and vegetables.
- Eat fat from avocados, coconut, and olive oil.
- Eat low glycemic fruits and non-starchy vegetables.
- Eat fermented foods like sauerkraut, coconut kefir, and yogurt.
- Eat Superfoods on a daily basis.
- Eat fiber from fruits and vegetables.
- Eat colorful veggies.
- Drink 8 glasses of water including veggie or bone broth daily.
- Exercise every day, preferably for 30 minutes.
- Meditate for at least 5 minutes per day.
- Take daily detox baths with Epsom salts, and baking soda.
- Drink green smoothies daily.
- Get 7-9 hours of sleep.
- Consider digestive enzymes, hydrochloric acid, and apple cider vinegar.

Don'ts:

- No grains at all.
- No dairy products
- No genetically modified organism (GMO) foods.
- No processed foods.
- No refined sugars.
- No wine or alcohol.
- No cereals or grain like seeds.
- No smoked or salted foods.
- No ibuprofen, aspirin or acetaminophen, naproxen.
- No legumes (e.g
- peanuts, beans, lentils, peas, and soybeans).
- No nuts, seeds or seed based spices.
- No nightshade vegetables.
- No fruit juices.
- No skipping meals.

Foods to Include:

FRUITS

Apples, apricots, Asian pears, bananas, blueberries, blackberry, boysenberry, cherries, cranberry, figs, grapefruit, kiwi, lemons, limes, melons, nectarine, oranges, peaches, pears, persimmons, plums, pluots, plantains, pomegranate, raspberry, strawberry

Caution: watermelon, mango, pineapple, grapes, dried fruits, dehydrated fruits.

VEGETABLES

Asparagus, arugula, artichoke, avocado, basil, beet, beet greens, broccoli, broccoli rabe, burdock, bok choy, cabbage, carrots, cauliflower, celery, chard, chicory, collards, chard, cucumber, scallion, Jerusalem artichoke, jicama, kale, kohlrabi, lambsquarters, leeks, lettuce, mustard, nettles, okra, onions, purslane, spinach, summer squash, turnips, artichoke hearts, Brussels sprouts, daikon radish, zucchini, fennel root, dandelion greens, red cabbage, green cabbage, Napa cabbage, water chestnuts, watercress, radish, shallot, turnips.

DENSE CARBS

Beets, acorn squash, butternut squash, yams, sweet potato, taro, plantain and lotus root.

FUNGI

Button mushrooms, portabella, oyster, chanterelle, puffball, crimini, etc.

WILD FISH

Salmon, mackerel, herring, halibut, shellfish, oysters, cod, tuna, flounder, sardines, hake, skate, trout, red snapper, etc.

MEAT

Beef, chicken; quail, squab, duck, goose, turkey, Cornish game hen; pasture-raised lamb, pork, buffalo/bison, goat, emu, ostrich, sausage (without fillers or nightshade spices); liver, kidney, heart, organic sliced meats (gluten, sugar free), uncured nitrate/nitrite-free deli meats and bacon from grass-fed/pastured beef/pork.

MILK AND YOGURT

Coconut milk, unsweetened coconut yogurt.

FATS

Extra virgin olive oil, coconut oil, flaxseed, sesame, walnut, hazelnut oil, coconut oil, red palm oil.

Caution: nut and seed based oils: flaxseed oil, sesame oil, walnut oil, hazelnut oil, macadamia nut oil.

COCONUT

Coconut oil, coconut butter, coconut milk, coconut cream, unsweetened coconut yogurt, unsweetened coconut flakes, coconut aminos, coconut kefir.

BEVERAGES

Filtered or distilled water, herbal tea, mineral water, broths, freshly made veggie juice, green smoothies, kombucha, kefir water, coconut kefir.

TEAS

Herbal teas: Peppermint, ginger, lemongrass, spearmint, chamomile, rooibos, lavender, cinnamon, milk thistle.

FERMENTED FOODS

Sauerkraut, pickles, pickled ginger, pickled cucumbers, unsweetened coconut yogurt, unsweetened coconut kefir (without corn or rice-based thickening agents), kombucha, kimchee, kefir water, pickles fermented with salt, beet kvass, lacto-fermented vegetables and fruits such as fermented beets, carrots, and green papaya.

CONDIMENTS

Apple cider vinegar, Balsamic vinegar, coconut vinegar, Red Boat fish sauce and coconut aminos.

HERBS AND SPICES

Turmeric, ginger, rosemary, basil, cilantro, garlic, ginger, lemongrass, peppermint, oregano, parsley, sage, sea, salt, thyme, tarragon, spearmint, marjoram, mace, chives, chamomile, chervil, cinnamon, bay leaves, cloves, dill, horseradish, saffron, sea salt.

Caution: black pepper, allspice, white, green and pink peppercorns, juniper, cardamom, star anise and vanilla bean.

SUGAR SUBSTITUTES

Cinnamon, mint and ginger

Caution: honey, maple syrup, molasses, unrefined cane sugar, and date sugar.

Foods to Eliminate:

NIGHTSHADE VEGETABLES

This includes potatoes (not sweet potatoes), all tomatoes, red and green peppers, chili peppers, eggplants, tomatillos, sweet bell peppers, jalapenos, cayenne, Habanero, Anaheim and Serrano et all peppers.

Avoid chili peppers in dried powders such as paprika, chili powder, curry powder, chili pepper flakes, hot sauces, Tabasco sauces, salsas, goji berries and ashwaganda.

FRUIT

Avoid canned fruits.

Caution: watermelon, mango, pineapple, grapes, dried fruits and dehydrated fruits.

PROCESSED AND CANNED MEATS

Bacon, fatty cuts of lamb, beef, pork, deli meats, smoked/dried/salted meat and fish. Sausages and deli meats with seed-based or nightshade spices.

FISH

Whale, shark, swordfish. Farmed tilapia and catfish quantities should be moderate.

NUTS AND SEEDS

Avoid all nuts and seeds including almonds, Brazil nuts, cashews, chestnuts, hazelnuts, macadamias, pecans, walnuts, pine nuts, pistachios, pumpkin, and sunflower seeds and seed based spices: anise, annatto, black cumin, celery, coriander, cumin, dill, fennel, fenugreek, mustard, nutmeg, poppy, sesame.

DAIRY

Cow and other animal (goat/sheep) milks, cheese, cottage cheese, cream, butter, yogurt, ice-cream, non-dairy creamers, soy milk, whey, butter, cheeses, frozen desserts, mayonnaise.

OILS

Margarine, butter, shortening, any processed hydrogenated oils, peanut oil, mayonnaise.

BEANS AND LEGUMES

Avoid-all beans, black-eyed peas, cashews, chickpeas, lentils, miso, peas, peanuts/peanut butter, soybean and soy products.

FUNGI

Avoid medicinal mushrooms e.g Shiitake, Maitake and Reishi mushrooms.

SOY

Soy milk, soy sauce, tofu, tempeh, soy protein, edamame.

DRINKS

Sodas, fruit juice, alcoholic beverages, coffee, green, black tea, all caffeinated beverages.

CONDIMENTS

Ketchup, relish, soy sauce, BBQ sauce, chutneys, other condiments, baker's and brewer's yeast.

SWEETENERS

Avoid white or brown sugar, high fructose corn syrup, corn syrup, fruit sweeteners, Truvia, maple syrup, agave, brown rice syrup, Splenda, Equal, Nutrasweet, Xylitol, stevia, raw green stevia.

GRAINS

Amaranth, barley, buckwheat, corn including cornmeal and popcorn, millet, oats, oatmeal, quinoa, rice, rye, sorghum, teff, triticale, and wheat including varieties such as spelt, emmer, farro, einkorn, kamut, durum and other forms such as bulgur, cracked wheat and wheat berries.

GRAIN PRODUCTS

Corn tortillas, chips, starch, syrup, noodles, cakes, breads, rolls, muffins, noodles, crackers, cookies, cake, doughnuts, pancakes, waffles, pasta, tortillas, pizza, pita, flat bread.

GRAIN LIKE SUBSTANCES OR PSEUDO-CEREALS

Amaranth, buckwheat, cattail, chia, cockscomb, kañiwa, pitseed, goosefoot, quinoa, and wattleseed (aka acacia seed).

GLUTEN CONTAINING FOODS

BBQ sauce, binders, bouillon, brewer's yeast, cold cuts, condiments, emulsifiers, fillers, gum, hot dogs, hydrolyzed plant and vegetable protein, ketchup, soy sauce, lunch meats, malt, malt flavoring, malt vinegar, matzo, modified food starch, monosodium glutamate, non-dairy creamer, processed salad dressings, seitan, stabilizers, teriyaki sauce, textured vegetable protein.

LEGUMES

Including peas, beans, lentils, soy, and peanuts.

LECTINS

Avoid nuts, beans, soy, potatoes, tomato, eggplant, peppers, peanut oil, peanut butter, soy oil, etc.

DAIRY

All dairy products, including milk cream, cheese, from cows, goats, sheep, etc.

EGGS:

Or foods that contain eggs (e.g mayonnaise).

ALCOHOL

All alcohol.

ALL PROCESSED FOOD

Cured meats, sugar, pre-mixed seasonings and sauces, mayonnaise, mustard, canned foods.

SUGARS

Avoid: white or brown sugar, high fructose corn syrup, corn syrup, fruit sweeteners, Truvia, agave, brown rice syrup, Splenda, Equal, Nutrasweet, Xylitol, stevia, raw green stevia, coconut sugar and palm sugar.

SEeD BASED SPICES

Anise, annatto, black cumin, celery, coriander, cumin, dill, fennel, fenugreek, mustard, nutmeg, poppy, sesame, cacao.

BERRY AND FRUIT BASED SPICES

Black pepper, allspice, white, green and pink peppercorns, juniper, cardamom, star anise and vanilla bean.

COFFEE

Remove coffee for 30 days, reintroduce and note reactions.

TEA

Remove caffeinated teas for 30 days, reintroduce and note reactions.

AVOID IMMUNE STIMULANTS

Echinacea purpurea extract, astragalus, ashwaganda, beta glucans, chlorella, glycyrrhiza, licorice root, goldenseal, panax ginseng, grape seed extract, Melissa officinalis (lemon balm), Maitake, Reishi, Shiitake, caffeine, green tea, coffee, lycopene, pine bark extract, willow bark, pycnogenol, genistein, quercetin.

A WORD ABOUT CAUTION FOODS

Generally speaking, these foods are either immunogenic, hard to digest, likely to feed gut bacterial overgrowths, dysbiosis, and/or contribute to blood sugar imbalance.

If your gut immunity is strong (no overgrowths, no dysbiosis, no food reactions, healthy gut lining), and your blood sugar is balanced, these items may be tolerated in moderation.

Considerations:

FODMAPs

Describe short-chain carbohydrates found in many common foods. FODMAPs stands for Fermentable Oligo-, Di- and Mono-saccharides, and Polyols (sugar alcohols).

FODMAP intolerance can tip you off to the possibility of having small intestine bacterial overgrowth If poorly digested, these carbs will feed bad bacteria (SIBO), which in turn produce methane and hydrogen gas that can cause bloating, cramping, burping, gas, diarrhea and other bowel problems that generally get diagnosed as IBS. If these bacterial overgrowths remain untreated, they may contribute to leaky gut and the inflammatory/immune response.

If you have IBS symptoms and are not improving on the standard Autoimmune Protocol, the best way to check for FODMAP sensitivity would be to remove these foods for at least 30 days and then reintroduce them and check for SIBO if there is no change.

If you desire to reintroduce these foods, make sure you have resolved the root cause of your FODMAP intolerance to avoid symptoms.

FODMAPs IN THE AIP

Apples, artichokes, apricots, cherries, pears, plum, persimmon, nectarines, peaches, pluots, artichoke, asparagus, cabbage, garlic, leeks, okra, onions, radicchio, avocado, beet root, broccoli, Brussels sprouts, mushrooms, butternut squash, pumpkin, cauliflower, celery, fennel bulb, mushrooms, sauerkraut, dried coconut, coconut flour, coconut milk, coconut cream, coconut butter, honey, grapes, dried fruits, blackberries, apricots, shallots.

SIBO CAUTION FOODS IN THE AUTOIMMUNE DIET

Parsnips, yams jicama, kohlrabi, okra, sweet potato, taro, plantain, Jerusalem artichoke, parsnips, lotus root, cassava root, manioc, tapioca, yucca.

Reintroduction of Foods:

Eliminate any foods on the "include" list that you suspect are problematic and do not agree with your constitution. For those not improving on *the standard* AIP and for those considering reintroduction of foods, it's important to be aware of the foods, herbs and compounds that may contribute to your symptoms and/or autoimmune reactions.

These include FODMAPs, starchy foods that contribute to SIBO, foods that create an antibody response (food sensitivities), high oxalate, high histamine and high salicylate foods, cross reactive proteins and immune stimulating herbs and compounds.

Since reintroduction of foods may cause pronounced reactions, it's important to inform your medical practitioner about your diet and about reintroducing foods and any exacerbation of symptoms.

When reintroducing a food, do so one food at a time, wait 72 hours, note any reactions (headache, joint ache, skin rash, decreased mental clarity etc.), wait until the symptom subsides, then reintroduce the next food.

AVOID IMMUNE STIMULANTS:

Echinacea purpurea extract, astragalus, ashwaganda, beta glucans, chlorella, glycyrrhiza, licorice root, goldenseal, panax ginseng, grape seed extract, Melissa officinalis (lemon balm), Maitake, Reishi, Shiitake, caffeine, green tea, coffee, lycopene, pine bark extract, willow bark, pycnogenol, genistein, quercetin.

Delicious Recipes:

GREEN SMOOTHIES

- 1/2 a bunch dino kale or swiss chard, cut out stalks
- 1/2 inch ginger
- ½ cup blueberries
- 5 cups of water

Blend for 5 minutes

VEGGIE STEW

- 1 and ½ cups water, divided
- 4 cups sliced onion
- 2 cups thinly sliced leek
- 1 1/2 cups (1/2-inch-thick) sliced carrots
- 3 cups (1-inch) cubed daikon (about 1 pound)
- 1 bay leaf
- 4 cups (1-inch) cubed zucchini (about 1 1/2 pounds)
- 1/2 teaspoon ground cinnamon
- dash of saffron
- 4 garlic cloves, minced
- 6 cups chopped Swiss chard (about 12 ounces)
- 1/2 cup chopped cilantro
- 2 1/2 teaspoons salt, divided
- 2 tablespoons fresh lemon juice

Add all ingredients to a crock pot or slow cooker

Cook on high heat for 2-3 hours.

COCONUT YOGURT

1. Heat 1 quart of unsweetened coconut milk to 105F - 110F.
2. Add ¼ teaspoon of yogurt starter and pulse 2x with the blender.
3. You can add more than 1/4 teaspoon per quart if a very firm yogurt is desired.
4. Plug in your yogurt maker and pour the mixture into your yogurt maker container or containers and ferment for 12 hours.
5. Place in refrigerator for 4 hours.

Enjoy with blueberries.

KALE CHIPS

Servings: 4.

- 1 large bunch of dino kale, stems removed and leaves chopped
- extra virgin olive oil
- sea salt to taste

Massage Kale with olive oil, sprinkle with sea salt and bake at 350 for 15 min. Let cool and give thanks for a great snack!

GRILL PAN CHICKEN

Servings: 2.

- 6 collard leaves, cut lengthwise into two large pieces (stems removed)
- carrot, cucumber, celery, cut into sticks
- handful of cilantro, whole or chopped
- avocado, sliced into wedges
- 2 organic chicken breasts coated with olive oil thyme and sea salt

Grill chicken, cut into slices and make a wrap with crunchy veggies inside the collard greens.

TRI-TIP STEAK AND ASPARAGUS

Servings: 3

- Tri-tip steak (1 pound)
- 1 head of asparagus
- olive oil
- sea salt
- 2 sprigs of fresh rosemary

Coat everything with olive oil, chopped rosemary, and salt. Grill to perfection.

COCONUT CHICKEN PAILLARD

Servings: 5.

- 5 chicken breasts
- salt to taste
- 1/2 cup coconut flour
- 3 TB olive or coconut oil
- 1 cup chicken broth
- 3 TB capers, drained and rinsed
- 4 sprigs fresh thyme

Coat chicken with olive oil, and salt. Then dip in coconut flour. Transfer chicken in a single layer to hot skillet and cook chicken cutlets 3 or 4 minutes on each side with capers and thyme. Add broth and cook for 15 minutes.

Serve.

BRAISED GREENS

Servings: 4.

- 2 TB coconut or olive oil

- 2 heads of greens
- 1/2 yellow onion, chopped
- 3 garlic cloves, chopped
- 1 1/2 cup vegetable, chicken, or beef stock
- salt to taste
- 2 TB apple cider vinegar

Sautee onion and garlic until golden brown then add greens, salt and vinegar. Cover and let the greens cook down for 20 minutes.

CARMELIZED BRUSSELS SPROUTS

Servings: 4.

- 1 lb Brussels sprouts
- 3 TBS balsamic vinegar
- 3 TBS olive oil

Sautee sprouts in olive oil on low heat until tender.

Increase to high heat and add balsamic vinegar, stir for 30 seconds, turn off flame and season with salt to taste.

BAKED TILAPIA WITH LEMON AND FRESH HERBS

Servings: 4.

- 1 shallot, finely chopped
- 4 tilapia fillets
- 4 teaspoons olive oil
- sea salt
- 1 teaspoon finely chopped fresh thyme leaves
- ½ TBSP chopped parsley
- ½ TBSP fresh cilantro
- 1 teaspoon salt
- finely grated zest of 2 lemons

Mix herbs and seasonings with olive oil. Add Lemon zest and spread half of seasoning over fish. Place fish in broiler pan lined with parchment paper. Broil in pre-heated broiler for 3 minutes. Turn fish, applying remaining seasoning and broil for 3-5 minutes

Serve.

SUPER GREENS SALAD

- 1 cup butter lettuce
- 1 cup spinach
- 1/2 cup dino kale (shredded)
- 1/4 cup parsley
- 1/8 cup fresh basil
- 1/8 cup carrots (diced or shredded)
- 1/8 cup celery (diced)

GINGER AVO COCO DRESSING

- 1/2 cup coconut or olive oil
- 1/3 cup raw apple cider vinegar
- 1/4 cup coconut aminos
- 1/2 cup water
- 2 tablespoon fresh ginger, grated
- 1 avocado

Blend and dress your salad!

BASIC BEEF BONE BROTH

- 4 quarts water
- 2 lbs beef bones (or oxtail)
- 6 garlic cloves
- 3 ribs of celery
- 1 onion chopped
- 2 tablespoon apple cider vinegar
- 1 teaspoon sea salt

Preparation:

1. Place all ingredients in pot and bring the stock to a boil, then reduce the heat to low and allow the stock to cook from 8 hours.
2. Strain to discard bones etc. Store your stock in the fridge and use within a few days.

GINGER ROOT TEA:

- 4-6 cup filtered water
- 2 tab freshly grated ginger root
- 1 Tbsp fresh lemon juice

Preparation

Bring ginger almost to boiling in the water. Turn off heat and let sit for 5-10 min. Add lemon juice and strain into a cup. You can reuse the ginger more than once by adding more water and heating.

ARUGULA SALAD WITH GRILLED TRI TIP

- 4 cups fresh arugula ½ Beet and 1 carrot peeled and grated
- 2 Tbsp olive oil
- 2 Tbsp balsamic vinegar
- Sea salt to taste
- ½ pound Tri-tip steak

Preparation

1. Mix arugula with grated beets, carrots in a large bowl.
2. Stir in the olive oil, vinegar, salt, and Adjust seasonings.
3. Sprinkle salt on Tri-Tip steak and cook on grill pan for 7-10 minutes on each side.

Servings: 1-2

PAN SEARED YELLOWTAIL WITH SAUTEED RAINBOW CHARD

- 1 pound yellow tail
- 2 Tbsp olive oil
- 1 bunch of chard
- 2 Tbsp coconut aminos
- 1 Tbsp minced ginger
- Sea salt to taste

Preparation

1. Marinate yellowtail ginger, coconut aminos and olive oil for 1 hour.
2. Sautee spinach in olive oil with salt to taste.
3. Spray and preheat skillet on med-high for 3 minutes.
4. Add yellow tail and cook for one minute per ½ inch of thickness, serve.

CHICKEN VEGETABLE SOUP

- 1 container chicken broth
- 1 grilled and sliced chicken breast
- ½ head of Dino Kale
- 2 Tbsp olive oil
- 1 sliced carrot
- ¼ bunch cilantro
- Sea salt to taste

Preparation

1. Sautee kale and carrot in olive oil.
2. Stir in the chicken broth, add salt, sliced chicken and cilantro.

Servings: 1-2

TUNA STEAKS WITH SAUTEED SPINACH

- 1 bunch washed spinach
- 1 pound Tuna Steaks
- 2 Tbsp coconut oil
- Sea salt to taste

Preparation

1. Wash, cut and sauté spinach in olive oil, sea salt to taste.
2. Coat Tuna steaks with olive spray, wasabi powder and sea salt
3. Grill for 5 minutes on each side

Servings: 1-2

NEW YORK STEAK AND SALAD

- 1 pound New York Steak
- 2 heads of washed romaine
- ½ cup grated Jicama plus 1 carrot peeled and grated
- 1 avocado
- 2 Tbsp olive oil
- 2 Tbsp apple cider vinegar
- Sea salt to taste
- olive oil spray

Preparation

1. Mix romaine with grated jicama, avocado, and carrots in a large bowl.
2. Stir in olive oil, vinegar, and salt.
3. Sprinkle sea salt and spray olive oil on New York Steak, cook on grill pan for 7 minutes per side. Slice and serve over salad.

Servings: 2

STEAMED HALIBUT WITH SAUTEED GREENS

- 1 pound halibut
- 1 inch of sliced ginger
- ¼ bunch cilantro
- 2 Tbsp coconut oil
- 2 tbsp coconut aminos
- Sea salt to taste
- One bunch of mustard greens

Preparation

1. Cover Halibut with coconut oil, coconut aminos, cilantro and ginger.
2. Steam the fish for 15 minutes.
3. Sauté mustard greens in olive oil, add salt to taste.

Servings: 2

STIR FRIED CHICKEN BREAST WITH ZUCCHINI, AVOCADO AND BASIL

Lettuce wrap

- 2 chicken breast
- 1 avocado sliced
- 3 medium zucchinis
- 1 bunch of basil
- 4 Tbsps olive oil
- olive oil spray
- Sea salt to taste
- 1 head of butter leaf lettuce

Preparation

1. Cut chicken into cubes and sauté in olive oil, pinch of salt.
2. After 5 minutes add zucchini in olive oil with basil.
3. Fill butter leaf lettuce with sauté and then add sliced avocado on top.

Servings: 2

TURMERIC CHICKEN WITH ZUCCHINI

- 2 chicken breast
- 3 medium zucchinis
- ¼ bunch of parsley
- 2 Tbsp olive oil
- 2 tsp Turmeric
- Olive oil spray
- Sea salt to taste

Preparation

1. Coat the chicken with olive oil spray, a light dusting of salt and turmeric. Grill for 8-10 minutes on each side.
2. Sautee zucchini in olive oil, parsley.
3. Slice the chicken and serve with sautéed zucchini.

Servings: 2

ROSEMARY BAKED LAMB CHOPS ON A BED OF KALE CHIPS

- 1 pound lamb chops
- 2 Tbsp minced fresh rosemary
- 2 teaspoons sea salt
- 2 Tbsp olive oil, divided
- 5 pieces of Kale
- Olive oil spray
- 1 Tbsp
- balsamic vinegar

Preparation

1. Rub chops with olive oil, rosemary and sea salt.
2. Spray olive oil in a baking dish.
3. Coat 5 large kale leaves with olive oil.
4. Place lamb chops on top of Kale.

5. Bake in oven @ 375F for 20 minutes, turn chops over, and cook for 20 more minutes, or to desired doneness.
6. Be sure to eat the kale chips!

Servings: 2-3

BALSAMIC MARINATED PORK CHOPS WITH MASHED TURNIPS AND SAUTEED COLLARDS

- 1 teaspoon sea salt
- 1/4 cup balsamic vinegar
- 6 Tbsp olive oil divided
- 2 bone in one pork chops
- 1 bunch of collard greens
- 4 turnip, boiled
- Sea salt to taste
- 4 turnips, boiled and mashed

Preparation

1. Marinate chops for at least one and up to 24 hours in balsamic vinegar and 2 Tbsp olive oil.
2. Grill 7 minutes per side, checking for doneness.
3. While turnips are boiling, sauté the collard greens in olive oil.
4. Mash turnip, add a dash of olive oil and salt to taste.

CROCK POT CHICKEN

- lbs boneless, skinless chicken thighs
- 3 parsnips, chopped
- 2 cloves of garlic
- ½ onion, chopped
- 3 carrots, chopped
- 4 celery stalks
- Sea salt to taste
- 2 medium zucchinis chopped
- 1/4 cup olive oil

- 1 TB dried thyme
- 1 TB sage
- 1 1/2 cups chicken broth

Preparation

Add everything to your slow cooker or crock pot and let cook on medium-high for 4 hours.

GRILL PAN PORK CHOPS

- 2 Pork Chops
- ¼ bunch of thyme
- Olive oil spray
- 1/8 Tsp sea salt to taste

Preparation

1. Mix thyme with olive oil and salt to rub chops.
2. Grill on med-high heat for 5-7 minutes per side.

Servings: 2

Preparation

Marinate mackerel in coconut aminos, olive oil and wasabi powder.

Grill for 5 minutes on each side.

Sautee spinach in olive oil, sea salt to taste.

Servings: 1-2

ZUCCHINI PASTA WITH SEASONED GROUND BEEF

- 2 large zucchinis, julienned
- ½ pound ground beef
- 2 cloves garlic, minced
- ¼ bunch chopped fresh basil
- ¼ bunch chopped fresh oregano
- Sea salt to taste
- Tbsp olive oil

Preparation

1. Sautee basil, garlic, oregano and beef in olive oil until fully cooked, add salt to taste.
2. Pour on top of zucchini pasta; add more fresh basil, Enjoy!

Servings: 1-2

BACON WRAPPED CHICKEN THIGHS

- 4 pieces of boneless, skinless chicken thighs
- 4 pieces of bacon
- 3 Tbsp olive oil
- 1 tsp sea salt

Preparation

1. Preheat the oven to 375 F
2. Coat chicken with olive oil and salt, fold in half then wrap one piece of bacon around each chicken thigh.
3. Bake for 30 minutes. Broil the chicken for another 5-10 minutes or until the bacon is crispy and the chicken is fully cooked.

ROSEMARY RUBBED CORNISH HENS

- 2 Cornish Hens (approx 1 lb
- each)
- 1 Tbsp olive oil
- 1 lemon wedge
- ¼ Tsp Sea salt
- 3/4 bunch of fresh rosemary, chopped
- ¼ bunch rosemary set aside for cavity

Preparation

1. Preheat oven to 450F.
2. Rinse hen, pat dry then rub with blend of oil, salt, chopped rosemary.

3. Place 1 lemon wedge and 3 sprigs of rosemary in cavity of each hen.
4. Put in roasting pan and cook at 450F for 25 minutes
5. Reduce heat to 350.
6. Mix chicken broth, and remaining 2 tablespoons of oil; pour over hens.
7. Continue roasting about 25 minutes longer, or until hens are golden brown.
8. Cut hens lengthwise and serve.

GROUND TURKEY BREAKFAST SAUTEE

- ½ pound ground turkey
- 1 Tbsp coconut aminos
- ½ onion
- 1 Tbsp minced garlic
- 2 large carrots, peeled and diced
- Sea salt
- 2 Tbsp olive oil
- 7 water chestnuts

Preparation

1. Sautee turkey in olive oil with coconut aminos, garlic, carrot, water chestnuts.
2. Add salt to taste, serve.

AHI TUNA WITH SAUTEED RED CHARD

- 1 one pound Ahi tuna steak
- 1 Tbsp coconut aminos
- 1 Tbsp minced ginger
- 4 Tbsp olive oil, divided
- 1 bunch red chard, chopped

Preparation

1. Marinate ahi in 2 Tbsp olive oil, coconut aminos and ginger for 1 hour or longer.
2. Sautee red chard in 2 Tbsp olive oil.

3. Grill tuna for 6 minutes each side or to desired doneness.

CARROT GINGER SOUP

- 7 large carrots, peeled and sliced thin
- Sea salt
- 1 teaspoon minced ginger
- ½ onion, chopped
- 2 cups of chicken or vegetable stock
- 2 cups water
- 3 large strips of zest from an orange
- Chopped parsley, dill and bacon for garnish

Preparation

1. Sautee carrots, ginger and onion in olive oil.
2. Add stock, water, ginger and orange zest.
3. Bring to a simmer, cover and cook for 20 minutes.
4. Remove orange zest strips.
5. Pour soup in a blender and puree until smooth.
6. Add salt to taste and garnish with bacon, parsley and dill.

Servings 4-5

GRASS FED BEEF BURGER

- ½ pound ground beef
- Sea salt to taste

Preparation

1. Add salt to ground beef and grill 2 burgers for 7 minutes on each side.
2. Optional: Top with bacon.

Servings:2

TRI TIP WITH SAUTEED GREENS AND MASHED CAULIFLOWER

- 1 pound Tri-tip steak
- 1 bunch of collard greens, rolled then cut thin
- 5 Tbsp olive oil
- Sea salt to taste
- 1 head of cauliflower

Preparation

1. Lightly salt Tri-tip and grill for 7 minutes on each side.
2. Sautee collard greens in olive oil.
3. Sprinkle salt on Tri-Tip and cook on grill pan.
4. Steam or pressure cook the cauliflower then mash and drizzle with olive oil.

Servings: 1-2

GRILLED CHICKEN BREAST WITH BRIGHT GREEN OLIVES

- 2 chicken breasts
- 20 bright green olives, pitted and chopped
- 3 Tbsp olive oil
- Fresh thyme leaves for 3 sprigs
- Olive oil spray

Preparation

1. Coat the chicken with olive oil spray, salt and thyme.
2. Heat oil on medium-high heat.
3. Add olives to the pan and sauté, and then cover sliced chicken with the sauce

RIB EYE STEAK WITH SAUTEED SWISS CHARD AND SWEET POTATO FRIES

- 1 pound skirt steak
- 1 bunch of Swiss Chard, chopped
- 5 Tbsp olive oil
- Sea salt to taste

Preparation

1. Lightly salt rib eye steak and grill for 10 minutes on each side.
2. Sautee chard in olive oil, serve.

Servings: 2

SWEET POTATO FRIES

- 3 medium sweet potatoes, washed and peeled
- 3 Tbsp coconut or olive oil
- 1 Tbsp salt or to taste

Preparation

Coat sweet potatoes with oil, salt

Spread on a baking sheet and bake at 425 for 20 minutes.

Servings: 4.

PACIFIC SNAPPER WITH LEMON, THYME AND CAPERS

- 1 1/2 pounds fresh Petrale sole fillets
- Approximately 40 capers
- 2 Tbsp olive oil
- Fresh thyme leaves
- Lemon wedges

Preparation

1. Pat the fish fillets dry with paper towels. Lightly salt the fillets on both sides.

2. Heat oil on medium-high heat. Brown the fillets gently on both sides for no more than a few minutes on each side.
3. Add capers to the pan and sauté with herbs, and a squeeze of lemon juice into the sauce. Drizzle sauce over fish.

Enjoy!

CHICKEN STOCK

- 2 ½ pounds bony chicken pieces
- 2 peeled and chopped carrots
- 1 peeled and chopped daikon
- 3 celery stalks
- 2 cloves of garlic
- ½ onion, chopped
- 2 bay leaves
- 2 quarts of water
- Sea salt to taste
- ¼ bunch fresh thyme leaves

Preparation

1. Add veggies, chicken and herbs to 2 quarts of water in a large pot.
2. Cook for 2 hours. When cool, discard.

SHRIMP SAUTEED WITH BOK CHOY

- 1/2 cup

GRILLED BALSAMIC PORK TENDERLOIN

Servings: 6.

- 8 garlic cloves, coarsely chopped
- 1 tablespoon fresh oregano, finely chopped
- 1 tablespoon fresh thyme, finely chopped
- 1 tablespoon fresh rosemary, finely chopped

- 1 teaspoon salt
- 1/4 cup balsamic vinegar
- 1/2 cup olive oil
- 2 one pound pork tenderloins

Marinade pork for up to 24 hours in above ingredients.

Grill to perfection. Serve.

CILANTRO ROAST CHICKEN

Servings: 2-4.

- 1 whole chicken, 6 lbs.
- 1 lime, juiced
- 1/2 bunch cilantro
- 3 green onions, chopped
- 6 cloves garlic, peeled
- 1/4 cup olive oil
- 1 TBSP coconut oil
- salt

Chop and mix ingredients, rub chicken

Bake at 400 for 45 minutes.

GARLIC ROSEMARY SALMON

Servings: 2.

- 2 salmon fillets
- 5 cloves garlic, crushed
- olive oil - enough to coat the salmon
- dried rosemary to taste
- the juice from 1 lemon

Mix garlic with dill, olive oil, lemon and coat the salmon. Grill pan to perfection.

BEEF STEW

Servings: 4-6

- grass-fed beef brisket 3 Lbs.
- 10 garlic cloves, peeled
- salt to taste
- 1 bay leaf
- 1 ½ cups beef broth
- 8 cups of veggies leeks, carrots, celery, onions

Cut slits into beef and add a peeled garlic clove in each. Sprinkle salt on beef. Chop up your veggies and add all ingredients to the slow cooker. Set on high for 4 hours or low for 8 hours.

SAUTÉED KALE

Servings: 4.

- 2 bunches of kale, leaves pulled off, discard stems
- 2 cloves garlic, finely chopped
- 1 TB olive oil

Sautee garlic in olive oil until golden brown, add in kale until tender.

GINGER SALMON AND BROCCOLI

Servings: 4.

- 1 head broccoli, cut into florets
- 2 TB coconut oil
- Sea salt
- 1-pound salmon
- Squeeze of lemon
- ¼ bunch fresh cilantro
- 1 TBSP ginger, chopped
- 2 TBS coconut aminos

Cover salmon with coconut oil, cilantro, ginger, coconut aminos and a squeeze of lemon. Grill pan to perfection and serve with steamed broccoli.

NORI CHIPS

Servings: 1.

- 3 Nori sheets
- Olive oil
- Sea salt

Preheat oven to 350

Cut Nori sheets into four and place on baking sheet. Brush or massage Nori with oil. Add sea salt and whatever spices you choose. Bake for 15 minutes.

Let cool.

PORTERHOUSE STEAK WITH KALE AND AVOCADO

- One 1 pound porterhouse steak
- 4 cups Russian red Kale
- 4 Tbsp olive oil
- Olive oil spray
- Sea salt to taste
- One avocado sliced on top of Kale

Preparation

1. Sautee kale in 4 Tbsp olive oil, sea salt to taste.
2. Sprinkle sea salt on meat and spray with olive oil.
3. Cook on grill pan for 10 minutes per side or to desired doneness.
4. Add avocado slices.

Servings: 2

SPAGHETTI SQUASH WITH GROUND TURKEY, GREENS AND ARTICHOKE HEARTS

- One medium spaghetti squash
- 4 cups packed spinach
- 7 artichoke hearts
- 5 Tbsp olive oil, divided
- ½ pound ground turkey meat
- 1 tsp dried oregano,
- 1 tsp dried basil
- Sea salt to taste

Bacon?

Preparation

1. Sauté spinach in 2 Tbsp olive oil until wilted, then add artichokes for 5 minutes and set aside.
2. Cut the spaghetti squash in half from top to bottom.
3. Remove the seeds from the middle of the squash
4. Place squash in a steamer for 20 minutes.
5. Add olive oil and oregano in medium sized skillet on med-high. Place the ½ pound of ground turkey in the skillet, breaking pieces apart. Make sure turkey is thoroughly cooked then add in bacon.
6. Once squash is tender, allow it to cool enough to remove insides of the squash. After all of the squash has been removed, place it in the skillet and mix together with turkey, bacon and greens.

Servings: 2

LEMON ORANGE CLAY POT CHICKEN

- One 3 pound chicken
- Juice of 1 lemon
- 1 blood orange, cut in half
- 3 Tbsp olive oil
- 5 sprigs of thyme, leaves pulled and chopped
- 6 cloves of garlic, chopped
- 5 sprigs of thyme for inside cavity
- 1 Turnip cubed
- 2 carrots, peeled and cut in quarters
- 1 Tbsp coconut aminos
- Sea salt to taste

Preparation

1. Soak clay pot roaster in cold water for 15 minutes.
2. Mix thyme, lemon juice, olive oil, garlic and coconut aminos.
3. Rinse chicken, pat dry then rub with salt, thyme and olive oil mix.
4. Cut turnips and carrots, coat with olive oil, sea salt to taste.
5. Place chicken on top of veggies in clay pot.
6. Squeeze the juice of one blood orange on top of chicken and veggies then place in cavity with lemon and thyme.
7. Cover clay pot and place in cold oven.
8. Raise temp to 400F and bake for 75 minutes, making sure chicken is cooked.

DESSERTS

COCONUT BERRY ICE CREAM

- 1 pint of blueberries or your favorites
- 1/2 cup coconut milk
- 1 tsp vanilla extract

Blend everything in your food processor and place in freezer.

RASPBERRIES WITH COCONUT MILK AND BALSAMIC VINEGAR

- 40 raspberries
- 2 Tbsp balsamic vinegar
- Coconut milk

Preparation

Cover raspberries in a bowl with 2 TBS of balsamic and let sit for 15 minutes. Drizzle with coconut milk.

SNACK IDEAS:

- Cucumber with sea salt
- Herbal tea
- Mixed fruit
- Coconut milk smoothie with plum, nectarine, peach, apple
- Nori Chips
- Kale Chips
- Coconut water kefir
- Coconut yogurt
- Avocado with sauerkraut
- Grated, Carrot, Daikon with Nori
- Bone Broth
- Veggie Broth

DETOX SUPPORT: TRANSITIONING TO THE AUTOIMMUNE DIET

Detox Bath Recipe:

- 2 pounds of Epsom Salts plus
- 1 pound of baking soda

DETOX BROTH:

- 3 quarts of water
- 1 large chopped onion
- 2 sliced carrots
- 1 cup of daikon
- 1 cup of turnips and rutabaga cut into large cubes
- 2 cups of chopped greens: kale, parsley, beet greens, collard greens, chard, dandelion, cilantro or other greens
- 2 celery stalks
- ½ cup of cabbage
- 4 ½ inch slices of ginger
- 2 cloves of whole garlic sea salt to taste

Preparation

1. Add all the ingredients at once and place on low boil for 60 minutes.
2. Cool and strain veggies out-discard them.

Makes approximately 8 cups. Store in fridge. Heat and drink 3-4 cups/day.

Additional Detox Support

LIVER DETOX:

Olive oil & lemon juice (one tablespoon of each mixed with 4 oz of water). Take one dose in morning and one in evening.

RAW APPLE CIDER VINEGAR:

1 tablespoon diluted with 1 tablespoon water helps your stomach produce hydrochloric acid, and aid digestion of proteins.

REDUCING STRESS AND IMPROVING SLEEP

Exercising for 30 minutes every day is ideal for enhanced sleep, immune modulation and stress reduction. I also recommend short daily meditation, acupuncture treatments, and massage for enhanced health.

Final Thoughts

The current recommendation among practitioners trained by Dr Kharrazian is at least a 45-day commitment to The Autoimmune Diet. Most patients will start noticing results sooner but 45 days is a necessary jumpstart to heal your leaky gut. Start by following the lists in this book regarding which foods to eliminate and include. Then find a practitioner to monitor your blood work and at a minimum, consider:

1. Supporting regulatory T-cells with: EPA/DHA, Probiotics, Vitamin D, and via supporting Glutathione: NAC, Alpha lipoic acid, L-glutamine, Milk Thistle, Cordyceps, Centella Asiatica, and Selenium

2. Clearing Dysbiosis and SIBO with: antimicrobial, anti-parasitic and/or anti-fungal botanicals and/or pharmaceuticals.

3. Supporting the integrity of the gut lining with: L-Glutamine, quercitin, zinc, DGL, aloe, and probiotic foods.

4. Adding digestive enzymes and hydrochloric acid for gas and bloating

5. Taking a multi/vitamin mineral, extra magnesium, Vitamin A, C and D. Get your D levels checked first.

6. Reduce inflammation with curcumin, resveratrol, Huperzine A, Vinpocetine, Adenosine, Alpha GPC, Xanthinol niacinate, and L- acetylcarnitine.

7. Support detoxification and methylation with folate, B6 and B12.

About the Author

Anne Angelone, Licensed Acupuncturist

Bachelor of Science, Cornell University Master of Science, American College of Traditional Chinese Medicine

Member of Primal Docs The Paleo Physician's Network

And Dr. Kharrazian's Thyroid Docs

✦ Background ✦

My own experience with Ankylosing Spondylitis (AS) led me to study the underlying mechanisms of disease expression. Since Ankylosing Spondylitis is correlated with the gene type called HLA B-27, I learned how to identify and remove specific triggers and then how to heal my leaky gut. I also learned how it's possible to turn off inflammatory gene expression with nutrition, supplements, Qi (oxygen), acupuncture, exercise, diet, and meditation. I'm grateful to be able to share what I have learned through experience and years of research, training and investigation.

My background in Functional Medicine has included advanced training with Dr. Datis Kharrazian in Functional Blood Chemistry Analysis, Mastering the Thyroid, Neurotransmitters and the Brain, Functional Endocrinology, Autoimmunity and Gluten Sensitivity

My hope is to share this information with those who would like to treat the underlying causes of "chronic symptoms" and experience greater health sooner than later.

For colorful food charts and a quick reference of FODMAP and SIBO foods, please check out my other e-book which is also available in paperback via createspace: *The Autoimmune Paleo Protocol*

For more info contact: www.anneangelone.com

AUTOIMMUNE PALEO RESOURCES:

Sarah Ballantyne, Ph.D aka: The Paleo Mom

Autoimmune and You

Autoimmune-Paleo Cookbook

Practical Paleo by Diane Sanfilippo

And Balanced Bites

Chris Kresser's: Personal Paleo Code

The Paleo Parents Pinterest page

Please check out Sarah Ballantyne's, book The Paleo Approach: Reverse Autoimmune Disease and Heal Your Body due to be in print in the very near future.

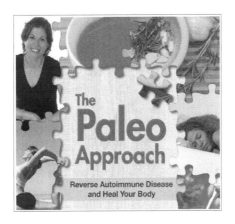

Made in the USA
San Bernardino, CA
07 March 2014